Defining High-Quality Care for Posttraumatic Stress Disorder and Mild Traumatic Brain Injury

Proposed Definition and Next Steps
for the Veteran Wellness Alliance

CARRIE M. FARMER, LU DONG

Sponsored by the George W. Bush Institute

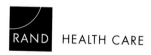

RAND HEALTH CARE

For more information on this publication, visit www.rand.org/t/RRA337-1

Library of Congress Cataloging-in-Publication Data is available for this publication.
ISBN: 978-1-9774-0589-0

Published by the RAND Corporation, Santa Monica, Calif.
© Copyright 2020 RAND Corporation
RAND® is a registered trademark.

Cover image: Bush Institute/Layne Murdoch, used with permission

www.rand.org

Preface

The Veteran Wellness Alliance, an initiative of the George W. Bush Institute, aims to connect post-9/11 veterans with peer networks and high-quality care for "invisible wounds," including posttraumatic stress disorder and mild traumatic brain injury. To further its mission, the Veteran Wellness Alliance asked the RAND Corporation to develop a definition of high-quality care for these conditions. This document describes the proposed definition and recommended next steps for implementing it.

This research was funded by the George W. Bush Institute and carried out within the Quality Measurement and Improvement Program in RAND Health Care.

RAND Health Care, a division of the RAND Corporation, promotes healthier societies by improving health care systems in the United States and other countries. We do this by providing health care decisionmakers, practitioners, and consumers with actionable, rigorous, objective evidence to support their most complex decisions. For more information, see www.rand.org/health-care, or contact

RAND Health Care Communications
1776 Main Street
P.O. Box 2138
Santa Monica, CA 90407-2138
(310) 393-0411, ext. 7775
RAND_Health-Care@rand.org

Contents

Tables

Abbreviations

APA	American Psychological Association
CAHPS	Consumer Assessment of Healthcare Providers and Systems
CBT	cognitive behavioral therapy
CPG	clinical practice guideline
CPT	cognitive processing therapy
DoD	U.S. Department of Defense
EMDR	eye movement desensitization and reprocessing
GAD-7	Generalized Anxiety Disorder–7-item
IOM	Institute of Medicine
IOP	intensive outpatient program
mTBI	mild traumatic brain injury
PCL-5	PTSD checklist for the *Diagnostic and Statistical Manual of Mental Disorders*, 5th edition (DSM-5)
PE	prolonged exposure
PHQ-9	Patient Health Questionnaire–9-item
PTSD	posttraumatic stress disorder
SSRI	selective serotonin reuptake inhibitor
TBI	traumatic brain injury
VA	U.S. Department of Veterans Affairs
VHA	Veterans Health Administration

Background

Many U.S. military veterans who served in the era after September 11, 2001, have experienced mental health problems, such as posttraumatic stress disorder (PTSD), and chronic issues resulting from traumatic brain injuries (TBIs) that occurred during their military service. These conditions, sometimes referred to as "invisible wounds," cause suffering for veterans and their families and can interfere with veterans' ability to work and contribute to their communities (Tanielian and Jaycox, 2008; Trivedi et al., 2015). Although there are effective treatments for these conditions, many post-9/11 veterans have had difficulty accessing high-quality care.

The George W. Bush Institute, a nonpartisan public policy arm of the George W. Bush Presidential Center, recognized the need to improve veterans' access to treatment and established the Veteran Wellness Alliance in 2017 (George W. Bush Institute, undated). As part of its mission, the Veteran Wellness Alliance connects post-9/11 veteran peer networks, which are organizations that provide support to veterans through social connection and a shared sense of purpose, with high-quality clinical care providers. The Veteran Wellness Alliance is composed of seven veteran peer network organizations and nine clinical partners, including the Veterans Health Administration (VHA), that collectively serve millions of post-9/11 veterans.

The Veteran Wellness Alliance and other veteran-serving organizations have a common goal to improve access to high-quality care for invisible wounds, but there is no shared definition of *high-quality care* to guide these improvement efforts. Establishing a clear standard for high-quality care would allow the Veteran Wellness Alliance to provide meaningful guidance to its clinical partners and the peer networks that help veterans access care. A definition of high-quality care for PTSD and TBI is also important for the broader community that serves post-9/11 veterans because it can set expectations for veterans seeking care for these conditions. Programs that provide care could also incorporate the definition into their strategic planning and quality improvement initiatives.

Veteran Wellness Alliance

Clinical Partners

- Cohen Veterans Network
- Emory Healthcare Veterans Program*
- Home Base, Massachusetts General Hospital and the Red Sox Foundation*
- Marcus Institute for Brain Health, University of Colorado Anschutz Medical Campus
- Operation Mend, University of California, Los Angeles*
- Road Home, Rush Medical Center*
- SHARE Military Initiative at Shepherd Center
- VHA

Peer Network Partners

- George W. Bush Institute Team 43
- Student Veterans of America
- Team Red, White, and Blue
- Team Rubicon
- The Mission Continues
- Travis Manion Foundation
- Wounded Warrior Project

* Member of the Wounded Warrior Project's Warrior Care Network (see Wounded Warrior Project, undated).

NOTE: See the appendix for additional information about Veteran Wellness Alliance clinical partners.

The Bush Institute asked the RAND Corporation to develop and implement a research-based and consensus-approved definition of high-quality care for invisible wounds, focusing specifically on PTSD and TBI. This document describes our approach to developing the definition and our recommendations for how the proposed definition could be used to improve care for veterans with PTSD and TBI.

Methods

To develop the definition of high-quality care, we first conducted an environmental scan of the research literature on health care quality, PTSD, and TBI, looking specifically for publications on the treatment of these conditions among veterans. We also reviewed clinical practice guidelines for PTSD and TBI, as well as reports and databases describing existing quality measures for these conditions. We used the findings from this environmental scan to draft a notional definition of high-quality care that spanned three components of care associated with positive outcomes for veterans with PTSD and TBI: veteran-centered care, evidence-based care, and measurement-based care.

Next, we conducted semistructured interviews with members of the leadership teams (e.g., medical director, chief of staff) of eight of the nine Veteran Wellness Alliance clinical partner organizations and four veteran peer network partner organizations, as well as one veteran family member/caregiver.[1] During each interview, we requested feedback on the notional definition and probed about aspects of care for PTSD and TBI that are perceived to be most important to the veterans served by these organizations. In interviews with clinical partners, we also gathered structured information about the veteran population served by the program, the types of care provided, and the types of patient outcome data that are routinely collected by the program.

We synthesized findings from the environmental scan and semi-structured interviews to refine the definition of high-quality care,

---

[1] We were unable to conduct an interview with one clinical partner because the timing of our interview coincided with the COVID-19 pandemic.

which we describe in detail here. We also present an example of how metrics could be used by the Veteran Wellness Alliance to identify programs that provide high-quality clinical care. We conclude this report with several recommended next steps for implementing and disseminating the proposed definition of high-quality care for veterans with PTSD and TBI.

What Does *Quality* Mean in the Context of Health Care?

Although there are multiple ways to define quality in health care, the definition proposed by the Institute of Medicine (IOM) in its groundbreaking report *Crossing the Quality Chasm* has been widely adopted (IOM, 2001a).[2] In this definition, *quality* is the degree to which health services for individuals and populations increase the likelihood of desired health outcomes and are consistent with current professional knowledge (IOM, 2001a). Health care quality, by this definition, can be measured across six key domains: patient-centeredness, timeliness, effectiveness, equity, safety, and efficiency (Table 1). Our definition of high-quality care for PTSD and TBI was adapted from this widely accepted definition.

Based on our review of the literature and interviews with Veteran Wellness Alliance clinical partners and peer network partners, we propose that a definition of high-quality care for invisible wounds include four components: care should be *veteran-centered, accessible,* and *evidence-based* and include *outcome monitoring.* We adapted the IOM definition of quality to encompass several aspects of care that are important to veterans. In particular, we expanded the IOM domain of patient-centered to be *veteran-centered,* including both the notion that care should be responsive to patient preferences and the uniqueness of veterans' experiences. We also expanded the IOM domain of timeliness to include other aspects of health care accessibility (e.g., "the five As" of accessibility: affordability, availability, accessibility, accommodation, and acceptability; see Penchansky and Thomas, 1981).

---

[2]   In March 2016, the Institute of Medicine was renamed the National Academy of Medicine and is part of the National Academies of Science, Engineering, and Medicine.

Table 1
IOM Definition of High-Quality Health Care

Domain	Definition
Patient-centered	Providing care that is respectful of and responsive to individual patient preferences, needs, and values and ensuring that patient values guide all clinical decisions
Timely	Reducing waits and sometimes harmful delays for both those who receive and those who give care
Effective	Providing services based on scientific knowledge to all who could benefit and refraining from providing services to those who are not likely to benefit (avoiding underuse and misuse, respectively)
Equitable	Providing care that does not vary in quality because of personal characteristics, such as gender, ethnicity, geographic location, and socioeconomic status
Safe	Avoiding harm to patients from the care that is intended to help them
Efficient	Avoiding waste, including waste of equipment, supplies, ideas, and energy

SOURCE: Adapted from IOM, 2001a.

We focused on evidence-based care and outcome monitoring as the critical components of the domains of effectiveness and safety for the purposes of our definition. We did not explicitly include the domain of equity because the objective of having a standardized definition is to ensure that all veterans receive high-quality care, regardless of their circumstances or geographic location. Finally, we did not include the domain of efficiency. We acknowledge that there might be a trade-off between efficiency and other aspects of high-quality care, but our definition does not address this.

Proposed Definition of High-Quality Care for Invisible Wounds

Veteran-Centered Care

The first pillar of high-quality care is grounded in the IOM's definition of patient-centered care. Patient-centeredness requires establishing a "partnership among practitioners, patients, and their families (when appropriate) to ensure that decisions respect patients' wants, needs, and preferences and that patients have the education and support they require to make decisions and participate in their own care" (IOM, 2001b, p. 7). Similar to a model of patient-centered care, the goals of veteran-centered care are to provide effective and timely care that addresses the unique needs, values, and preferences of veterans. In particular, providing veteran-centered care requires that health care providers be attentive to the exposures and implications of prior military service. Effective veteran-centered care is achieved through a combination of military cultural competency, patient-centered communication, and clinical acumen (Hamm et al., 2008). Our proposed definition of veteran-centered care is described in Table 2.

> **High-quality care** for invisible wounds should be
>
> **veteran-centered**
> **accessible**
> **evidence-based.**
>
> It should also include
> **outcome monitoring.**

Table 2
Defining Veteran-Centered Care

Aspect of Veteran-Centered Care	Description
Provides culturally competent care	Staff members are trained in and provide culturally competent care, including military cultural competence and across several domains of diversity (e.g., gender, race/ethnicity).
Assesses veteran experience of care	Program regularly solicits information (e.g., via patient surveys) about veterans' satisfaction with care, perceived ability to access care, perception of provider communication, and other aspects of the patient experience.
Includes shared decisionmaking	Program includes the veteran in all treatment decisions and incorporates the veteran's preferences and unique circumstances in treatment planning. Ideally, program has a protocol for shared decisionmaking.
Involves family/caregivers	To the extent that the veteran desires, program includes family members/caregivers in treatment.

Summary of the Literature

Veteran-centered care is recommended by clinical practice guidelines (CPGs) developed by the U.S. Department of Veterans Affairs (VA) and U.S. Department of Defense (DoD) and mentioned as a key aspect of quality care for veterans in the research literature. As we explored the literature, we identified several key components to the concept of veteran-centered care.

First, because veterans' military experience plays an important role in both their health conditions and, for many, their identity, it is critical that health care providers who serve veterans receive training in military cultural competence (Meyer, Writer, and Brim, 2016). Military cultural competence includes providers' knowledge and comfort related to military culture (e.g., chain of command, military norms, military identity) and how it influences veterans' responses to illness (Meyer, Writer, and Brim, 2016). It also includes providers' attitudes toward veterans and skill sets to assess and treat service members and veterans (Atuel and Castro, 2018). Research has suggested that providers' military cultural competence may be a key factor in improving mental health care outcomes for veterans and their families (Tanielian et al., 2014).

In addition to military cultural competence, providers who work with veterans should also have cultural competence in other sociocultural dimensions underlying their patients' health beliefs and behaviors (e.g., gender, race/ethnicity). In general, providers' lack of culturally competent practices—stemming from a failure to acknowledge, understand, and manage sociocultural variations in the health attitudes and behaviors of their patients—is associated with poor communication with patients and problems with alliance formation. It could also lead to patient dissatisfaction, nonadherence to treatment, and worse health outcomes. However, research has yet to establish an empirical link between providers' cultural competence and improvements in patient-level health outcomes (Betancourt and Green, 2010; Horvat et al., 2014).

Second, similar to patient-centered care in general, veteran-centered care involves incorporating veterans' values and unique circumstances into clinical decisionmaking and engaging veterans in shared decisionmaking. Shared decisionmaking is an interactive process in which patients/clients and clinicians collaborate to share relevant information, enable patient-centered selection of health care resources, and make health care decisions (Adams and Drake, 2006). Research suggests that the majority of patients, including veterans seeking outpatient mental health care, prefer to be offered options, asked their opinions, and actively involved in the decisionmaking process (Park et al., 2014; Chewning et al., 2012).

Shared decisionmaking has been linked to some benefits, although there is still a lack of evidence establishing an empirical link between shared decisionmaking and patient behavior and health outcomes. For example, there is some evidence that shared decisionmaking may be particularly suitable for mental health care as an effective method to improve patient satisfaction, treatment adherence, and treatment outcomes (Joosten et al., 2008). There is also some evidence that shared decisionmaking tends to result in greater improvements in affective-cognitive patient outcomes (e.g., patient understanding, satisfaction, trust), compared with behavioral (e.g., treatment adherence, health behaviors) and health (e.g., symptom reduction, quality of life) outcomes (Shay and Lafata, 2015). In our definition, we suggest that it may be desirable to use a protocol for shared decisionmaking because prior evidence shows some effectiveness of using decision aids for improving patient outcomes (Stacey et al., 2017).

Finally, veteran-centered care should also include caregiver and family involvement, as desired by the veteran. This is consistent with the patient- and family-centered approach in which planning, delivery, and evaluation of health care is grounded in mutually beneficial partnerships among patients, families, and health care providers (Institute for Patient- and Family-Centered Care, 2016). Family-centered care models have been developed for pediatric care, critical care, and rehabilitation for stroke patients (Kokorelias et al., 2019). Several aspects of the family-centered care model appear to be suitable for veterans and their families. For example, the universal goal for family-centered care—regardless of the specific patient population—is to develop and implement care plans within the context of families.

Key components of a family-centered approach include patient and family education, collaboration between family members and health care providers, consideration of family contexts, and dedicated policies and procedures to support the implementation of a family-centered approach (Kokorelias et al., 2019). Although, to our knowledge, a family-centered care model has not been formally defined for veterans, there has been recognition of the importance of incorporating family-centered interventions into treatments for combat-injured veterans when family involvement is clinically indicated (Cozza et al., 2013). Such family-centered interventions may include such strategies as reducing family distress and disorganization, educating family members about the impact of the injury and the expected recovery process, and developing optimism and future hopefulness. Research also suggests that a substantial minority of veterans prefer to have family involved in their mental health care (e.g., to increase their education about the illness) (Cohen et al., 2019). We note that, although our interviewees acknowledged the importance of family involvement in veterans' health care, there appears to be limited research focused specifically on family-centered care for veterans.

Summary of Veteran Wellness Alliance Partner Interviews

All Veteran Wellness Alliance clinical partner programs reported providing veteran-centered care that maps to the components we identified through our literature review. For example, all programs reported that they required and provided training in cultural competence, particularly military cultural competence. Some programs indicated that they prioritize recruiting clinicians with prior training and experience with military populations.

Veteran Wellness Alliance clinical partners indicated that they actively engage patients in some level of shared decisionmaking, although there was no standard protocol across programs. Clinical partners described several practices that supported shared decisionmaking, including providing patient education (e.g., explaining evidence-based treatment, such as cognitive processing therapy [CPT]), using the client's language to describe treatment goals and to present problems, training clinicians in collaborative documentation and case conceptualization, building infrastructure for collaborative decisionmaking, offering optional care to individualize the treatment experience (e.g., acupuncture), and designating a primary provider to discuss individual needs. All the programs also reportedly involved family members and offered case management and follow-on care coordination.

During our interviews, Veteran Wellness Alliance clinical and peer partners shared feedback and suggested additions to our proposed definition of high-quality care. Many clinical and peer partners mentioned the importance of family/caregiver involvement and integration as a component of veteran-centered care. For example, some programs reportedly offered an optional family curriculum in parallel to treatment, focusing on psychoeducation on PTSD and treatment, as well as communication training. Several partners added that our proposed definition should acknowledge sustainability, citing the need for a healthy balance between high-quality care and its cost and the resources it requires. Finally, several clinical partners mentioned the need for broader cultural competence training for providers to be able to work with veterans with diverse backgrounds, including gender and race/ethnicity.

Accessibility

High-quality care is accessible and timely, meaning that veterans are able to obtain care without a long wait for an appointment. In addition, programs that provide high-quality care work to address and reduce geographic, financial, and other barriers. Improving veterans' access to care has been an intense focus in recent years, for both VA and other veteran-serving organizations. VA has established access standards for the care it provides to veterans, specifying both geographical access (how far veterans travel for care) and timeliness (how long veterans wait for an appointment), and it regularly monitors and publicly reports how well it is doing in meeting these standards (VA, undated). Veteran-centered and evidence-based care (as discussed later) have limited utility if veterans are unable to access care, making it critical for a definition of high-quality care to emphasize timeliness and accessibility. Our proposed definition of accessible care is described in Table 3.

Summary of the Literature

Accessibility of care is a multifaceted construct that can be described by "the 5 As of access": affordability, availability, accessibility, accommodation, and acceptability (Penchansky and Thomas, 1981). Studies have identified barriers to veterans' access to mental health care in each of these domains (Cheney et al., 2018; DeViva et al., 2016; Fox, Meyer, and Vogt, 2015; Garcia et al., 2014; Hoge et al., 2004). Veterans who are not eligible for VA health care may face financial barriers, and even those who *are* eligible may have concerns about cost or face related

Table 3
Defining Accessible Care

Aspect of Accessible Care	Description
Ensures that care is timely	Program has adequate appointment availability; veterans do not have to wait a long time after being referred to or requesting care.
Reduces barriers to care	Program considers potential geographic, financial, and cultural barriers to care and works to eliminate or reduce them (e.g., by providing care at no cost to veterans).

barriers due to lack of childcare or transportation (Garcia et al., 2014; Cheney et al., 2018). Veterans may not perceive care as accessible or acceptable due to perceived stigma, fear of repercussions or perceived career harms, a lack of confidence in navigating health care systems and services, or a belief that they can handle it on their own or that available treatments are not effective (Hoge et al., 2004; DeViva et al., 2016; Fox, Meyer, and Vogt, 2015). Veterans in rural areas or far from VA facilities may perceive care as less accessible, and there is evidence that rural veterans use less mental health care as a result (Teich et al., 2017).

Timeliness is an especially important dimension of accommodation, and one that has received significant attention from veterans, advocacy groups, and Congress (Hussey et al., 2015; IOM, 2014). Although this evidence is not specific to mental health care, long wait times and delayed access to necessary care can negatively affect health outcomes and patient satisfaction (Prentice and Pizer, 2007; Pizer and Prentice, 2011).

Summary of Veteran Wellness Alliance Partner Interviews

In terms of reducing personal, financial, and physical barriers to accessing high-quality care, all Veteran Wellness Alliance clinical partners reported offering treatment at no cost to the veteran. Although many programs collected insurance information from patients, across all programs, access to care was not limited by the ability to pay. Clinical partners that offered an intensive outpatient program (IOP) also reported providing transportation and lodging during the course of treatment. Some programs were considering or testing options to shorten the duration of their IOPs to further reduce potential barriers related to time commitment. In terms of providing timely care, all clinical partners indicated an intention to offer ready access to care. (Some programs were able to operate without a waiting list for eligible veterans; some also reported that they offered case management if ready access was not available.) Veteran Wellness Alliance peer network partners reported that, from their perspective, timely and easy access to care was the most important aspect of high-quality care for PTSD and TBI.

Evidence-Based Care

The third pillar of our definition aligns with the IOM's definition of safe and effective care. High-quality care is based on research evidence and adheres to clinical practice guidelines. The IOM defined evidence-based practices as the integration of the best research evidence with clinical expertise and patient values (IOM, 2001a). This definition has also been adopted by many professional societies; for example, the American Psychological Association (APA) has a very similar definition of evidence-based practice for psychology in which the integration of best available research and clinical expertise should occur "in the context of patient characteristics, culture, and preferences" (APA Presidential Task Force on Evidence-Based Practice, 2006).

Best available research evidence refers to scientific findings related to interventions, assessments, clinical problems, and patient populations in both laboratory and field settings, as well as clinically relevant results from basic research. For treatments or interventions, the best evidence comes from systematic reviews and randomized controlled trials. For other clinical questions, other types of evidence may be more suitable—for example, qualitative studies for understanding patient experiences and concerns, process-outcome studies for identifying mechanisms of change, or epidemiological data for understanding the prevalence of a clinical problem.

Clinical expertise is the "proficiency and judgment that individual clinicians acquire through clinical experience and clinical practice" (Sackett et al., 1996, p. 71). APA has specified several areas of clinical expertise for mental health providers:

> assessment, diagnostic judgment, case formulation, and treatment planning; clinical decision making, treatment implementation, and monitoring of patient progress; interpersonal expertise; continual self-reflection and acquisition of skills; appropriate evaluation and use of research evidence . . . ; understanding the influence of individual, cultural, and contextual differences on treatment; seeking available resources . . . as needed; and having a cogent rationale for clinical strategies. (APA Presidential Task Force on Evidence-Based Practice, 2006, p. 276)

Patients' unique values and circumstances, further specified by APA as patient characteristics, culture, and preferences in the context of psychological treatments, have gained greater emphasis since the first definitions of evidence-based practice in medicine (APA Presidential Task Force on Evidence-Based Practice, 2006; Sackett et al., 1996).

In our definition, providing evidence-based care means that there is a high concordance with clinical practice guidelines and updates from the best available research evidence (e.g., systematic reviews and meta-analyses). Our proposed definition of evidence-based care is described in Table 4.

Veteran Wellness Alliance clinical partners serve some veterans who have complex symptom presentations or have experienced treatment failures before. In these cases, there is room for innovation in treatment approaches while incorporating what is known from the best available research literature and clinical experience—an approach known as evidence-*informed* treatment. In general, however, evidence-based treatments and practices that follow established CPGs should be the primary basis of high-quality care for PTSD and TBI.

Table 4
Defining Evidence-Based Care

Aspect of Evidence-Based Care	Description
Performs a comprehensive assessment	Program performs structured clinical and diagnostic assessments to inform treatment.
Provides trauma-focused psychotherapy for PTSD	Program prioritizes individual, trauma-focused psychotherapy, such as prolonged exposure, CPT, eye movement desensitization and reprocessing (EMDR), or cognitive behavioral therapy (CBT).
Provides multidisciplinary team-based treatment for TBI	Program prioritizes symptom-driven care from a coordinated, multidisciplinary team that includes neurology, physical therapy, neuropsychiatry, and other specialties.
Performs appropriate screenings	Program performs risk screenings, including suicide and homicide risk, military sexual trauma, and unhealthy alcohol and drug use.
Includes care coordination and treatment planning	Program coordinates care with veterans' other providers and ensures treatment continuity.

Summary of the Literature on Evidence-Based Care for PTSD

Treatment of PTSD in veterans and adults is guided by several CPGs: VA/DoD (2017), APA (2017), World Health Organization (2013), International Society for Traumatic Stress Studies (2017), and the UK's National Institute for Health and Care Excellence (2018). CPGs are developed by a panel of multidisciplinary experts and based on a systematic review of clinical and epidemiological evidence.

Clinical guidelines recommend trauma-focused psychotherapy as a first-line treatment for PTSD. For example,

- Prolonged exposure
- Cognitive processing therapy
- Eye movement desensitization and reprocessing
- Cognitive behavioral therapy for PTSD
- brief eclectic psychotherapy
- narrative exposure therapy
- written narrative exposure.

There is consistency across these guidelines in the recommended care for PTSD. Specifically, trauma-focused psychotherapies received the highest overall recommendations across CPGs, and selective serotonin reuptake inhibitors (SSRIs) were recommended as the most effective medications (Hamblen et al., 2019). In addition, there is general consensus that trauma-focused psychotherapies should be offered as the first-line treatment for adults with PTSD, with or without medications. For example, the VA/DoD (2017) guideline recommends offering psychotherapy before medication, adding that medication should not be used in the absence of psychotherapy. The World Health Organization guideline recommends that medication treatments (e.g., SSRIs and tricyclic antidepressants) be considered when recommended psychotherapies have failed or are unavailable or when patients present with comorbid moderate to severe depression.

We provide a brief overview of the recommendations and suggestions from the VA/DoD and APA CPGs as they relate to the treatment of PTSD for veterans. The VA/DoD CPG recommends individual, manualized, trauma-focused psychotherapy over other pharmacologic and nonpharmacologic interventions as the primary treatment (VA/DoD, 2017). A primary component of this approach is exposure or cognitive restructuring and can include PE, CPT, EMDR, specific types of CBT for PTSD, brief eclectic psychotherapy, narrative exposure therapy, or written narrative exposure. When individual trauma-focused psychotherapy is not available or not preferred, the VA/DoD CPG recommends selected types of pharmacotherapy (e.g., sertraline, paroxetine, fluoxetine, venlafaxine) or individual non–trauma-focused psychotherapy (e.g., stress inoculation training), present-centered therapy, or interpersonal psychotherapy).

Consistent with the VA/DoD CPG, the APA CPG for treating adults with PTSD recommends trauma-focused psychotherapies with varying levels of strength and confidence (APA, 2017). Treatments with the strongest evidence that are most highly recommended are CBT, CPT, cognitive therapy, and PE therapy. In terms of comparative effectiveness, the guideline recommends that clinicians offer either PE or PE with cognitive restructuring when both are being considered. The guideline also suggests that clinicians offer CBT or PE rather than relaxation therapy when considering these options. Unlike the VA/DoD CPG, the APA CPG states that the strength of evidence is conditional for brief eclectic psychotherapy, EMDR, and narrative exposure therapy and that there is insufficient evidence for relaxation and the Seeking Safety treatment model. APA has suggested that its recommendations for EMDR and narrative exposure therapy are likely to change from "conditional" to "strong" in light of new evidence (APA, 2017).

A recent meta-analysis suggests that the best available evidence to date supports individual trauma-focused psychotherapy as the first-line psychological treatment of PTSD for active-duty military and veteran populations, although it found that the evidence for effectiveness in these populations was not as strong as it was for nonmilitary populations (Kitchiner et al., 2019). Other recent meta-analyses concluded that trauma-focused interventions were only marginally superior relative to non–trauma-focused approaches for treating military-related PTSD due to heterogenous outcomes and high nonresponse rates in the studies reviewed (Steenkamp et al., 2015; Steenkamp, Litz, and Marmar, 2020). More research is needed to investigate why some patients respond to trauma-focused interventions and others do not, as well as differences between military and nonmilitary populations. Additional research is also needed to determine how to best match patients to particular interventions and to develop and test new treatment approaches. Despite the need for additional research, the best available evidence and most current CPGs still suggest that providing high-quality care for PTSD involves offering individualized, trauma-focused psychotherapy as a first-line treatment.

Summary of the Literature on Evidence-Based Care for TBI

The VA/DoD CPG for mild TBI (mTBI, also known as a concussion) aims to assist providers in managing or co-managing adult patients with a history of mTBI (VA/DoD, 2016). It does not address individuals in the immediate period (within seven days) following mTBI, individuals with moderate or severe TBI, or children or adolescents. The VA/DoD CPG recommends evaluating individuals who present with symptoms or complaints potentially related to brain injury at initial presentation and suggests conducting a focused diagnostic assessment specific to any symptoms that develop more than 30 days after an mTBI. For co-occurring conditions, the CPG recommends assessing patients with symptoms attributed to mTBI for psychiatric symptoms and comorbid psychiatric disorders (e.g., major depressive disorder, PTSD, substance use disorder, suicidality).

In terms of treatment, the VA/DoD CPG suggests a primary care, symptom-driven approach to evaluating and managing patients with a history of mTBI and persistent symptoms. The CPG has specific guidance on managing such symptoms as sleep disturbance, headache, dizziness and disequilibrium, behavioral symptoms, cognitive symptoms, visual symptoms, and tinnitus (ringing in the ears). For patients with a history of mTBI and cognitive symptoms (those that do not resolve within 30–90 days and have been refractory to treatment for associated symptoms), the CPG recommends referral for structured cognitive or neuropsychological assessment to determine functional limitations and guide treatment. The CPG does not recommend conducting a comprehensive or focused neuropsychological assessment in the first 30 days after an mTBI or for *routine* diagnosis and care of patients with mTBI-related symptoms. The CPG also suggests that patients with mTBI and persistent or treatment-refractory cognitive symptoms (e.g., memory, attention, or executive function loss) be referred to a short-term cognitive rehabilitation therapist with TBI expertise.

Other expert consensus and practice guidelines indicate that managing mTBI involves regular symptom monitoring to inform adjustments to activity resumption (Lumba-Brown et al., 2018b; Marshall et al., 2018). Past expert consensus and practice guidelines for managing mTBI have recommended rest and patient education (see Farmer et al., 2016). Patients used to be advised to avoid physical activity, cognitively demanding tasks, and exposure to sensory stimuli until symptoms are completely resolved. However, recent evidence shows that a relatively prompt return to usual activities, as long as it does not exacerbate symptoms, may lead to faster recovery, while prolonged rest is associated with longer recovery and more symptoms (Lumba-Brown et al., 2018a; McCrory et al., 2017; Silverberg, Duhaime, and Iaccarino, 2020). Hence, the current recommendation is to monitor symptoms concurrently with a gradual return to activities. Neuroimaging should also be considered selectively (e.g., for those with life-threatening intracranial injury, alternation of consciousness, severe headaches, repeated vomiting, and/or seizures), but most patients do not need computed tomography imaging (Silverberg, Duhaime, and Iaccarino, 2020).

Although most adults with mTBI recover within one to three months, for some individuals, recovery can be slow and mTBI symptoms may be persistent. Psychiatric, psychological, or psychosocial factors (e.g., related to premorbid and injury-related emotional distress or life disruption), physical symptoms, and neurological factors can contribute to persistent mTBI symptoms (McCrory et al., 2017; Silverberg, Duhaime, and Iaccarino, 2020). Patients with persistent symptoms or those who are unable to return to activities should be referred to multidisciplinary centers for specialty care (McCrory et al., 2017; Silverberg, Duhaime, and Iaccarino, 2020).

Treatment for those with persistent symptoms related to mTBI is highly variable, depending on the patient's presentation, but the primary goal of treatment is to alleviate symptoms (Polinder et al., 2018). A meta-analysis showed little support for pharmacologic interventions for depression, anxiety, and mood problems related to mTBI, although some new evidence shows promising effects in using sertraline to prevent mood problems following TBI (Barker-Collo, Starkey, and Theadom, 2013; Jorge et al., 2016). Evidence regarding nonpharmacological interventions (e.g., psychoeducational interventions, cognitive/neuropsychological rehabilitation, such psychotherapeutic approaches as CBT, integrated behavioral health interventions for mTBI and PTSD) targeting persistent symptoms following mTBI is also limited (Barker-Collo, Starkey, and Theadom, 2013; Cooper et al., 2015). For example, research has found that the effect of CBT on symptoms related to mTBI was marginal, but CBT was associated with improved health-related quality of life as part of outpatient rehabilitation services (Potter, Brown, and Fleminger, 2016). Overall, despite limited evidence, a multidisciplinary assessment and treatment approach to addressing the complex etiology of persistent symptoms following an mTBI may be the most promising (Polinder et al., 2018).

Summary of Veteran Wellness Alliance Partner Interviews

In general, clinical partners reported that they prioritized providing evidence-based care. VHA has long been a leader in providing evidence-based care for PTSD and TBI (VA, 2019). Indeed, VHA has generated much of the evidence for the treatment of PTSD and TBI, as well as the clinical practice guidelines for treating these conditions.

All the other clinical partner programs for PTSD treatment reported that they prioritized individual psychotherapy over medication treatment, although they offered medication management if needed. The majority of clinical programs offered evidence-based treatments and made extensive efforts to ensure the fidelity of implementation, such as through formal training, regular supervision, or a review of treatment session recordings). All clinical partner programs described providing and requiring extensive didactic training on evidence-based psychotherapies, as well as ongoing supervision and consultation. Some clinical partners provided resources for clinicians to obtain certifications in certain psychotherapies (e.g., CPT, PE).[1] Some programs

---

[1] We note that training and certification programs vary in their ability to ensure competency in implementing evidence-based practices (Hepner et al., 2019).

reported allowing more innovation in terms of providing evidence-*informed* treatment for psychological conditions, depending on clinical experience and expertise, as well as unique patient characteristics.

Programs that focused on TBI treatment relied heavily on evidence-based, standardized assessment and a multidisciplinary team–based model in which each discipline adopts evidence-based approaches and care is tailored to veterans' specific deficits and needs.

Regarding our proposed definition of high-quality care, some clinical partners elaborated on the concept of evidence-based care and stated that it is important to recognize that high-quality care should be *responsible*: Treatment should be based on the best available evidence, and treatment gains should ideally be sustained when veterans return to their homes and lives. In addition, clinical partners indicated that treatment should not only incorporate the most effective evidence-based approach, but it should also be delivered with adequate competence and fidelity, although they acknowledged that it is difficult to measure treatment fidelity and ensure that delivery and implementation are effective.

Outcome Monitoring

The final pillar of our definition, outcome monitoring, is the routine administration of validated measurement tools, such as symptom rating scales, to assess and monitor clinical outcomes. Outcome monitoring can guide clinical decisionmaking and collaborative treatment planning with patients (Fortney, Sladek, and Unützer, 2015). VHA has been a leader in using data from outcome monitoring to provide measurement-based care, in which outcome data are shared with patients and used to inform treatment decisions. Through a multiphase effort that began in 2016, VHA has been attempting to increase adoption of measurement-based care in behavioral health across its health care system (VA, 2016). However, evaluations of this effort have shown significant challenges to adopting measurement-based care that may take time to overcome (Brooks Holliday et al., 2020). Implementing regular monitoring of clinical outcomes and effects on life and well-being—including functioning, life satisfaction, relationship quality, and the ability to return to work and reintegrate into civilian life—is a critical starting point (Table 5).

Summary of the Literature

There is increasing recognition of the importance of regularly measuring patient outcomes as a component of mental and behavioral health care (Fortney, Sladek, and Unützer, 2015). The use of measurement-based care in behavioral health has been required by the Joint Commission, a health care accreditation and certification body (Lavin, Berry, and Williams, 2017). Measurement-based care typically involves three main components: (1) collecting patient-reported data routinely throughout treatment, (2) using the information to inform treatment decisions, and (3) regularly sharing the information with patients to engage them in shared decisionmaking about their treatment and with the rest of the treatment team or administrators (Lewis et al., 2019; Wray et al., 2018). Outcome monitoring is also considered a core component of evidence-based practices (Beck, 2011; Klerman et al., 1984), and it is empirically supported as an evidence-based framework that can be added to any psychological treatment (Lambert et al., 2003). Outcome monitoring may include gathering information about symptoms, functioning and satisfaction with life, putative mechanisms of change (e.g., readiness to change), and the treatment process (e.g., session feedback, patient-provider relationship) (Scott and Lewis, 2015).

Table 5
Defining Outcome Monitoring

Aspect of Outcome Monitoring	Description
Monitors clinical outcomes	Program uses a validated instrument to regularly assess clinical outcomes (e.g., at treatment initiation and throughout treatment).
Monitors effects on life and well-being	Program uses a validated instrument to regularly assess aspects of well-being, such as functioning, relationship quality, and life satisfaction.

Evidence shows that outcome monitoring and measurement-based care are associated with increased quality and effectiveness of mental health care. At the patient level, measurement-based care involves sharing feedback on treatment progress and symptom severity levels with patients (Boswell, 2017), which allows patients to be more engaged in their treatment (Fortney, Sladek, and Unützer, 2015; Fortney et al., 2017). This measurement-based feedback intervention has been associated with better clinical outcomes in integrated primary care and specialty mental health care, as well as with preventing treatment failure in integrated primary care and outpatient specialty mental health care (Kearney et al., 2015; Knaup et al., 2009; Shimokawa, Lambert, and Smart, 2010).

Outcome monitoring is consistent with patient-centered care and can be used as a tool to engage patients in shared decisionmaking (Boswell et al., 2015; Santana and Feeny, 2014). Routine outcome monitoring promotes timely feedback on a patient's treatment progress and allows clinicians to identify patients who are not responding to treatment and are at risk of deteriorating (Boswell, 2017; Boswell et al., 2015). Outcome monitoring also supports data-driven clinical decisionmaking; if a patient is not responding to treatment, alternative courses of action may be considered, such as using a different medication or evidence-based treatment, or making appropriate referrals (Fortney et al., 2017; Kearney et al., 2015; Fortney, Sladek, and Unützer, 2015). At the system or organizational level, it can provide data for program evaluation and insight to support quality improvement (Fortney, Sladek, and Unützer, 2015; Kearney et al., 2015).

Summary of Veteran Wellness Alliance Partner Interviews

All Veteran Wellness Alliance clinical partner programs indicated that they monitor clinical outcomes, but VHA was the only clinical partner with a robust measurement-based care approach. In VHA's measurement-based care initiative, all sites use at least one core measure: PTSD Checklist for DSM–5 (PCL-5; Weathers et al., 2013), Patient Health Questionnaire–9-item (PHQ-9; Kroenke, Spitzer, and Williams, 2001), Generalized Anxiety Disorder–7-item (GAD-7;

Spitzer et al., 2006), or the Brief Addiction Monitor (Cacciola et al., 2013), which is administered at intake and at repeated predetermined intervals. Clinicians enter the data into VHA's electronic health record system and share the results with veterans during visits and with other providers as needed and as clinically appropriate for treatment planning (Brooks Holliday et al., 2020).

Each of the other programs reported performing an intake assessment to either confirm the diagnosis or refer the patient for a comprehensive evaluation for treatment planning purposes. Clinical partner programs reported using standardized assessment procedures to monitor clinical outcomes throughout treatment, with symptoms and functioning typically assessed with validated self-report measures and at multiple times during pretreatment, post-treatment, and follow-up (usually at one month or three months, six months, and 12 months). Some programs reported using outcome measures collected pre- and postintervention to define treatment response or success, as well as tracking outcomes during treatment to inform clinical decision-making. Programs also reported routinely screening for suicidality, homicidality, and unhealthy drug and alcohol use.

The four Warrior Care Network programs (Emory, Road Home, Operation Mend, and Home Base) offer two- to three-week IOPs to treat PTSD, TBI, and related conditions. These programs agreed to collect data from a set of common patient outcome measures, such as the PCL-5 for PTSD symptoms and the PHQ-9 for depression symptoms. We show in Table 6 an example of some of the measures collected by one Warrior Care Network program, Road Home at Rush University Medical Center. As a primary PTSD treatment program, Road Home defines treatment success as a reduction of ten points or more on the PCL-5.

Table 7 shows some of the outcome measures tracked by the Cohen Veterans Network, which provides brief outpatient evidence-based psychotherapy for depression, anxiety, and posttraumatic stress. The clinical outcome measures used are specific to the patient's symptoms. Table 8 presents some of the outcomes collected for inter-disciplinary evaluation and IOP treatment at the Marcus Institute for Brain Health, which provides comprehensive care for veterans with mTBI and PTSD, while Table 9 presents some of the outcomes collected by the SHARE Military Initiative at Shepherd Center, a comprehensive rehabilitation program focusing on assessment and treatment for mTBI. Note that these tables provide examples of the main measures tracked by different programs; they are not an exhaustive account of all data that these programs collect.

Table 6
Example of Patient Outcomes Collected at an Intensive Outpatient Program for PTSD Treatment: Road Home, Rush University Medical Center

		Data Collection Time Points			
Domain	Measure	Pretreatment	During Treatment	Discharge	Follow-Up[a]
Alcohol use	AUDIT-C	X		X	X
Anxiety	GAD-7	X	X	X	X
Depression	BDI	X		X	X
	PHQ-9[b]	X	X	X	X
Drug use screening	DAST-10	X			
Health-related quality of life	RAND-36	X		X	X
Illness severity (clinician)	CGI[c]		X		
Mindfulness	FFMQ	X			
Physical functioning	PROMIS SF 8a	X		X	X
PTSD diagnosis	CAPS	X			
PTSD symptoms	PCL-5[b]	X	X	X	X
Resilience	CD-RISC-10	X		X	X
TBI symptoms	NSI	X		X	X
Trauma-related guilt	TRGI[d]	X	X	X	X

Table 6—Continued

Domain	Measure	Data Collection Time Points			
		Pretreatment	During Treatment	Discharge	Follow-Up[a]
Trauma-related cognition	PCTI	x		x	
Vocational Needs/values	MIQ	x			
Personality traits	SD3	x			

NOTES: AUDIT-C = Alcohol Use Disorders Identification Test for Consumption scale. BDI = Beck Depression Inventory. CAPS = Clinician-Administered PTSD Scale. CD-RISC-10 = Connor-Davidson Resilience Scale. CGI = Clinical Global Impression scale. DAST-10 = Drug Abuse Screen Test. FFMQ = Five Facet Mindfulness Questionnaire. MIQ = Minnesota Importance Questionnaire. NSI = Neurobehavioral Symptom Inventory. PCTI = Posttraumatic Cognitions Inventory. PROMIS SF8a = Patient-Reported Outcomes Measurement Information System Short Form–Physical Function 8a. RAND-36 = RAND-developed 36-item measure of health-related quality of life. SD3 = Short Dark Triad personality measure. TRGI = Trauma-Related Guilt Inventory.

[a] Follow-up assessments conducted at three, six, and 12 months post-treatment.

[b] PHQ-9 and PCL-5 are given every other day to track depression symptoms and PTSD, respectively.

[c] CGI is rated by a clinician at every encounter during the treatment.

[d] During treatment, TRGI is given every day to track trauma-related guilt.

Table 7
Example of Patient Outcomes Collected at an Outpatient PTSD Program: Cohen Veterans Network

Domain	Measure	Referral Screener	Intake	Monthly	Every session	Termination
				Data Collection Timepoints		
Alcohol use	AUDIT-C	x				
Anxiety	GAD-7		x	x^a		x
Couple relationship	RDAS-1 (couples only)		x^b			
Depression	PHQ-9	x		x^a		x
PTSD	PC-PTSD	x				
	PCL-5		x^b	x^a		x^a
Quality of life, enjoyment, satisfaction	Q-LES-Q-SF	x		x		x
Substance use	CAGE-AID	x				
Suicide	C-SSRS			x	x^c	x
TBI screening	DVBIC	x	x			

NOTES: AUDIT-C = Alcohol Use Disorders Identification Test for Consumption scale. CAGE-AID = CAGE alcohol dependence questionnaire adapted to include other drugs. C-SSRS = Columbia-Suicide Severity Rating Scale. DVBIC = Defense and Veterans Brain Injury Center TBI screening tool. PC-PTSD = Primary Care PTSD Screen. Q-LES-Q-SF = Quality of Life Enjoyment and Satisfaction Questionnaire–Short Form. RDAS = Revised Dyadic Adjustment Scale.

[a] Completed for each diagnosis.

[b] Completed if indicated by the PC-PTSD.

[c] Completed if needed.

Table 8
Example of Patient Outcomes Collected at an Intensive Outpatient Program for TBI Treatment: Marcus Institute for Brain Health

Domain	Measure	Data Collection Time Points		
		Pretreatment Evaluation	Intake	Discharge and Follow-Up[a]
Anxiety symptoms	GAD-7	x	x	x
Cannabis use	DFAQ-CU	x	x	x
Client satisfaction	CSQ-8			x
Daytime sleepiness	Epworth Sleep Scale	x	x	x
Depression symptoms	PHQ-9	x	x	x
Dizziness	DHI	x	x	x
Fatigue	MFIS	x	x	x
Functional impairment	WHODAS 2.0	x	x	x
Global impression of change	PGIC			x
Impact of headache	HIT-6	x	x	x
Neurobehavioral symptoms	Neurobehavioral Checklist	x	x	x
Pain intensity	PROMIS-Pain	x	x	x
PTSD symptoms	PCL-5	x	x	x
Quality of life	RAND SF-36	x	x	x
Reasons for termination (RT)	RT-P[b] RT-T[b]	x	x	
Sleep quality and pattern	PSQI	x	x	x
Substance-related risk and problems	CRAFFT	x	x	x
TBI symptoms	NSI	x	x	x

Table 8—Continued

Domain	Measure	Pretreatment Evaluation	Intake	Discharge and Follow-Up[a]
		Data Collection Time Points		
Treatment credibility	Credibility scale		x	x
Treatment expectancy	Expectancy scale	x		

NOTES: CRAFFT = Car, Relax, Alone, Forget, Friends, Trouble (screen for substance-related risks and problems). CSQ = Client Satisfaction Questionnaire. DFAQ-CU = Daily Sessions, Frequency, Age of Onset, and Quantity of Cannabis Use Inventory. DHI = Dizziness Handicap Inventory. HIT = Headache Impact Test. MFIS = Modified Fatigue Impact Scale. NSI = Neurobehavioral Symptom Inventory. PGIC = Patient Global Impression of Change. PROMIS-Pain = Patient-Reported Outcomes Measurement Information System Pain Intensity Measure. PSQI = Pittsburgh Sleep Quality Index. RAND-36 = RAND-developed 36-item measure of health-related quality of life. RT-P = Reasons for Termination–Patient. RT-T = Reasons for Termination–Therapist. WHODAS = World Health Organization Disability Assessment Schedule.

[a] Follow-up time points are one, six, and 12 months post-discharge and annually thereafter.

[b] RT-P and RT-T are administered only in cases of early termination from the program.

Table 9

Example of Patient Outcomes Collected at an Intensive Outpatient Program for TBI Treatment: SHARE Military Initiative

Domain	Measure	Intake	Discharge	Follow-Up
		Data Collection Time Points		
Adaptability after TBI	MPAI-Adjustment	x	x	
	MPAI-Ability	x	x	
	MPAI-Participation	x	x	
Alcohol use	AUDIT	x		
Customer satisfaction	Customer satisfaction survey		x	
Depressive symptoms	BDI	x	x	
Dizziness	DHI	x	x	
Global functioning	GAS[a]	x	x	x
Impact of headache	HIT	x	x	
Insomnia symptoms	Insomnia Severity Index	x	x	
Life satisfaction	SWLS	x		
Pain	POQ	x	x	
PTSD symptoms	PCL-5	x	x	
Sleep quality and pattern	PSQI	x	x	
Suicide screening	C-SSRS	x		
Traumatic life events	Life Events Checklist	x		

NOTES: AUDIT = Alcohol Use Disorders Identification Test. BDI = Beck Depression Inventory. DHI = Dizziness Handicap Inventory. C-SSRS = Columbia-Suicide Severity Rating Scale. GAS = Global Assessment Scale. HIT = Headache Impact Test. MPAI = Mayo-Portland Adaptability Inventory. POQ = Pain Outcomes Questionnaire. PSQI = Pittsburgh Sleep Quality Index. SWLS = Satisfaction With Life Scale.

[a] GAS is administered at one, two, three, six, nine, and 12 months post-discharge. Additional measures (not shown in the table) for occupational therapy and physical therapy are administered at admission and discharge.

Operationalizing High-Quality Care: Potential Metrics

The proposed definition of high-quality care is comprehensive, encompassing multiple aspects of care for veterans with PTSD and TBI. As a next step, the Veteran Wellness Alliance will need to consider how to operationalize the definition: What is the best way to measure whether a clinical program is providing high-quality care?

Based on our review of the literature and existing measure repositories, we suggest several metrics of high-quality care as a starting point for further research (Table 10). Veteran Wellness Alliance clinical partners will need to provide input on the feasibility of collecting data to populate these indicators, and peer network partners and other stakeholders will need to provide guidance on the usability of the metrics for discerning whether a clinical program is providing high-quality care.

The suggested metrics cover all aspects of the high-quality care definition and would draw data from a variety of sources: patient surveys, program records, and patient medical records. All clinical partners currently conduct patient satisfaction surveys. It may be possible to include additional questions, such as those used in the Consumer Assessment of Healthcare Providers and Systems (CAHPS) surveys administered by the Agency for Healthcare Research and Quality, to report on veterans' care experiences in a way that could be compared across health care providers. VA's ongoing patient surveys are based on CAHPS. Data from medical records, needed to report on certain aspects of care, may or may not be available in comparable forms across Veteran Wellness Alliance clinical partners; for example, some clinical partners may already capture data on the type of psychotherapy received by veterans with PTSD, while others may only record that psychotherapy was received.

Table 10
Potential Metrics for High-Quality Care for Invisible Wounds

Measure	Component of High-Quality Care	Data Source	Measure Source
How well providers communicate with patients (composite patient experience measure)	Veteran-centered	Patient surveys	CAHPS
Program staff have received training in military cultural competence	Veteran-centered	Program records	RAND
Timely appointments, care, and information (composite patient experience measure)	Accessible	Patient surveys	CAHPS
New patients can schedule first appointment within 14 days of requesting care	Accessible	Program records	RAND
New patients assessed for PTSD/ TBI with validated instrument	Evidence-based	Medical records	Hepner et al., 2016
New patients assessed for suicide/ homicide risk with validated instrument	Evidence-based	Medical records	RAND
Patients with a history of mTBI receive multidisciplinary evaluation	Evidence-based	Medical records	RAND
Patients with PTSD receive trauma-focused psychotherapy	Evidence-based	Medical records	Hepner et al., 2016
Patients with PTSD receive weekly (or more frequent) psychotherapy visits	Evidence-based	Medical records	Hepner et al., 2016
Providers use validated instrument to assess patient symptoms and inform treatment	Outcome monitoring	Medical records	Hepner et al., 2016
Providers assess functional status using a validated instrument at least twice in the first six months of treatment	Outcome monitoring	Medical records	RAND

Recommendations

This report described our proposed definition of high-quality care for veterans with invisible wounds, specifically PTSD and TBI. Grounded in the IOM's definition of quality care, our definition posits that high-quality care is veteran-centered, accessible, and evidence-based and includes outcome monitoring. Based on a review of the literature and interviews with Veteran Wellness Alliance partners, we further specified key components of each of these pillars of high-quality care.

The following recommendations for the implementation and dissemination of this definition of high-quality care will help ensure broad uptake and improved support for veterans with PTSD and TBI.

Ensure That Necessary Data Are Available and Feasible to Report

Although we proposed a few potential metrics that the Veteran Wellness Alliance could use to operationalize the definition of high-quality care, additional work is required to assess whether these or other measures should be utilized. The Veteran Wellness Alliance should ask clinical partners what types of data are available and feasible to report. For example, can programs easily retrieve data from their medical records? Can they add questions to existing patient surveys? Upcoming working group meetings will provide some insights, but additional work will be required to determine how best to specify the measures, given data availability.

Develop an Implementation Plan

The Veteran Wellness Alliance should consider how it will use the high-quality care definition and associated measures. For example, will programs be required to report these quality measures, or will such reporting be voluntary? How often will it occur? How and where will the quality measure performance information be communicated to alliance member organizations and the public? If the definition is to be used to vet potential new clinical partners, what steps will those programs need to take to demonstrate that they provide high-quality care?

Develop a Dissemination Plan

The Veteran Wellness Alliance should drive quality standards and quality improvement for the broader clinical community that provides care to veterans with PTSD and TBI. It should set this bar and clearly declare what high-quality care means to its partners. Moving forward, the Veteran Wellness Alliance should promote the use of this definition throughout the veteran-serving community by working with peer network partners to disseminate and communicate information about high-quality care for veterans, through thoughtful engagement at stakeholder events and meetings, and by collaborating with other clinical providers on quality improvement initiatives.

Overview of Veteran Wellness Alliance Clinical Partners

Table A.1 presents additional information about Veteran Wellness Alliance clinical partners: their missions, the services and evidence-based treatments they provide, and an example outcome measurement for each.

Table A.1
Veteran Wellness Alliance Clinical Partners

Veteran Wellness Alliance Clinical Partners	Mission/Goal	Services Provided	Components of Evidence-Based Treatment	Example Outcome Measurement
Cohen Veterans Network[a]	Providing personalized, confidential, and genuine care to veterans; primary goal is to provide ready access to high-quality care	Brief outpatient psychotherapy for depression, anxiety, and posttraumatic stress	Individual CBT, CPT, PE, and CBT-i	Use CAPS to confirm diagnosis; use PCL-5, PHQ-9 and other validated measures to track psychological symptoms and functioning at multiple follow-ups; patient satisfaction survey
Home Base, Massachusetts General Hospital and the Red Sox Foundation[b]	Healing the invisible wounds of service members, veterans, and their families	2-week IOP and outpatient veteran and family clinic	• PTSD: evidence-based individual psychotherapy • mTBI: multidisciplinary treatment efforts, including appointments with physical medicine and rehabilitation, physical therapy, and meetings with neurology or neuroendocrine specialists, if appropriate	Use validated measures, such as PCL-5 and PHQ-9, to track symptom severity and functioning at multiple follow-ups; patient satisfaction survey
Emory Healthcare Veterans Program[b]	Working to get the member to the highest level of functioning following a recovery-based model	2-week IOP for PTSD, outpatient program, and family services	• Trauma-focused individual psychotherapy, including CPT and PE • DBT • Stress management • Sleep treatments	Use PCL-5, PHQ-9, AUDIT, CD-RISC-10, and other validated measures to track symptoms and functioning; patient satisfaction survey

Table A.1—Continued

Veteran Wellness Alliance Clinical Partners	Mission/Goal	Services Provided	Components of Evidence-Based Treatment	Example Outcome Measurement
Marcus Institute for Brain Health, University of Colorado Anschutz Medical Campus	Providing comprehensive care to benefit military veterans with a history of mTBI and PTSD	3-day interdisciplinary evaluation for mTBI and PTSD and 3-week IOP	• Individual psychotherapy (e.g., EMDR, CBT-i, CBT for chronic pain) • Physical therapy • Speech therapy	Use PCL-5, PHQ-9, PSQI, and other validated measures to track symptom severity and functioning; patient satisfaction survey
Operation Mend, University of California, Los Angeles[b]	Partnering with the U.S. military to jointly heal the wounds of war	3-week IOP plus 3-week telehealth peer support for PTSD, mTBI, and depression; outpatient mental health program for PTSD	• PTSD: individual CPT and group therapy (e.g., DBT skills, mindfulness) • mTBI: cognitive training, medication management	Use PCL-5, PHQ-9, and other validated measures to track symptom severity and functioning at multiple follow-ups (including in-person follow-up); patient satisfaction survey
Road Home, Rush Medical Center[b]	Providing psychotherapy-focused, evidence-based care for veterans with PTSD	3-week IOP (including individual and group therapy, options for medication management and TBI assessment/recommendations); outpatient care for local veterans	• Individual CPT • Mindfulness-based resiliency training • DBT skills coaching (for multisystemic therapy group)	Confirm PTSD diagnosis using CAPS; monitor symptom severity and functioning using validated measures (e.g., PCL-5, PHQ-9) at multiple follow-ups; patient satisfaction survey

Table A.1—Continued

Veteran Wellness Alliance Clinical Partners	Mission/Goal	Services Provided	Components of Evidence-Based Treatment	Example Outcome Measurement
SHARE Military Initiative at Shepherd Center	Providing a comprehensive rehabilitation program focused on assessment and treatment for mTBI	IOP for mTBI and co-occurring behavioral health concerns	• 1.5- to 2-week IOP for comprehensive evaluation for mTBI; most stay 4–12 weeks for treatment: • Individual sessions with physical, occupational, recreational, and speech therapists, physician, and nutrition/dietician • Individual and group psychotherapy for co-occurring mental health issues • Neuropsychological assessment if appropriate	Use MPAI and other validated measures to track adaptive living skills and functioning across multiple domains, as well as symptom severity and attainment of individualized client goals; patient satisfaction survey
VHA	Providing comprehensive health care services, including mental health care, to eligible military veterans	Comprehensive care for PTSD, other mental health disorders, and TBI, including outpatient psychotherapy, medication management, inpatient and residential treatment, IOPs, and rehabilitation	Numerous trauma-focused psychotherapies for PTSD and a full range of treatment for TBI	Use PCL-5, PHQ-9, and other validated measures to assess symptoms and functioning/quality of life/well-being; patient satisfaction survey

NOTES: CAPS = Clinician-Administered PTSD Scale. CBT-I = cognitive behavioral therapy for insomnia. DBT = dialectical behavior therapy. MPAI = Mayo-Portland Adaptability Inventory. PHQ9 = Patient Health Questionnaire-9. CD-RISC-10 = Connor-Davidson Resilience Scale. AUDIT = Alcohol Use Disorders Identification Test. PSQI = Pittsburgh Sleep Quality Index.

a Cohen Veterans Network consists of 19 outpatient clinics around the country; they may offer somewhat different services.

b Member of the Wounded Warrior Project's Warrior Care Network

References

Adams, Jared R., and Robert E. Drake, "Shared Decision-Making and Evidence-Based Practice," *Community Mental Health Journal*, Vol. 42, No. 1, February 2006, pp. 87–105.

American Psychological Association, *Clinical Practice Guideline for the Treatment of Posttraumatic Stress Disorder*, Washington, D.C., February 24, 2017.

American Psychological Association Presidential Task Force on Evidence-Based Practice, "Evidence-Based Practice in Psychology," *American Psychologist,* Vol. 61, No. 4, May–June, 2006, pp. 271–285.

APA—*See* American Psychological Association.

Atuel, Hazel R., and Carl A. Castro, "Military Cultural Competence," *Clinical Social Work Journal,* Vol. 46, No. 2, 2018, pp. 74–82.

Barker-Collo, Suzanne, Nicola Starkey, and Alice Theadom, "Treatment for Depression Following Mild Traumatic Brain Injury in Adults: A Meta-Analysis," *Brain Injury,* Vol. 27, No. 10, 2013, pp. 1124–1133.

Beck, Judith S., *Cognitive Behavior Therapy: Basics and Beyond*, 2nd ed., New York: Guilford Press, 2011.

Betancourt, Joseph R., and Alexander R. Green, "Linking Cultural Competence Training to Improved Health Outcomes: Perspectives from the Field," *Academic Medicine,* Vol. 85, No. 4, April 2010, pp. 583–585.

Boswell, James F., "Psychotherapy Integration: Research, Practice, and Training at the Leading Edge," *Journal of Psychotherapy Integration,* Vol. 27, No. 2, June 2017, pp. 225–235.

Boswell, James F., David R. Kraus, Scott D. Miller, and Michael J. Lambert, "Implementing Routine Outcome Monitoring in Clinical Practice: Benefits, Challenges, and Solutions," *Psychotherapy Research,* Vol. 25, No. 1, 2015, pp. 6–19.

Brooks Holliday, Stephanie, Kimberly A. Hepner, Carrie M. Farmer, Christopher Ivany, Praise Iyiewuare, Pearl McGee-Vincent, Shannon McCaslin, and Craig S. Rosen, "A Qualitative Evaluation of Veterans Health Administration's Implementation of Measurement-Based Care in Behavioral Health," *Psychological Services*, Vol. 17, No. 3, August 2020, pp. 271–281.

Cacciola, John S., Arthur I. Alterman, Dominick DePhilippis, Michelle L. Drapkin, Charles Valadez, Jr., Natalie C. Fala, David Oslin, and James R. McKay, "Development and Initial Evaluation of the Brief Addiction Monitor (BAM)," *Journal of Substance Abuse Treatment*, Vol. 44, No. 3, March 2013, pp. 256–263.

Cheney, Ann M., Christopher J. Koenig, Christopher J. Miller, Kara Zamora, Patricia Wright, Regina Stanley, John Fortney, James F. Burgess, and Jeffrey M. Pyne, "Veteran-Centered Barriers to VA Mental Healthcare Services Use," *BMC Health Services Research*, Vol. 18, No. 1, 2018, article 591.

Chewning, Betty, Carma L. Bylund, Bupendra Shah, Neeraj K. Arora, Jennifer A. Gueguen, and Gregory Makoul, "Patient Preferences for Shared Decisions: A Systematic Review," *Patient Education and Counseling*, Vol. 86, No. 1, January 2012, pp. 9–18.

Cohen, Amy N., Eric R. Pedersen, Shirley M. Glynn, Alison B. Hamilton, Kirk P. McNagny, Christopher Reist, Eran Chemerinski, and Alexander S. Young, "Preferences for Family Involvement Among Veterans in Treatment for Schizophrenia," *Psychiatric Rehabilitation Journal*, Vol. 42, No. 3, September 2019, pp. 210–219.

Cooper, Douglas B., Anne E. Bunner, Jan E. Kennedy, Valerie Balldin, David F. Tate, Blessen C. Eapen, and Carlos A. Jaramillo, "Treatment of Persistent Post-Concussive Symptoms After Mild Traumatic Brain Injury: A Systematic Review of Cognitive Rehabilitation and Behavioral Health Interventions in Military Service Members and Veterans," *Brain Imaging and Behavior*, Vol. 9, No. 3, September 2015, pp. 403–420.

Cozza, Stephen J., Allison K. Holmes, and Susan L. van Ost, "Family-Centered Care for Military and Veteran Families Affected by Combat Injury," *Clinical Child and Family Psychology Review*, Vol. 16, No. 3, September 2013, pp. 311–321.

DeViva, Jason C., Christina M. Sheerin, Steven M. Southwick, Alicia M. Roy, Robert H. Pietrzak, and Ilan Harpaz-Rotem, "Correlates of VA Mental Health Treatment Utilization Among OEF/OIF/OND Veterans: Resilience, Stigma, Social Support, Personality, and Beliefs About Treatment," *Psychological Trauma*, Vol. 8, No. 3, May 2016, pp. 310–318.

Farmer, Carrie M., Heather Krull, Thomas W. Concannon, Molly M. Simmons, Francesca Pillemer, Teague Ruder, Andrew M. Parker, Maulik P. Purohit, Liisa Hiatt, Benjamin Saul Batorsky, and Kimberly A. Hepner, *Understanding Treatment of Mild Traumatic Brain Injury in the Military Health System*, Santa Monica, Calif.: RAND Corporation, RR-844-OSD, 2016. As of September 8, 2020: https://www.rand.org/pubs/research_reports/RR844.html

Fortney, John, Rebecca Sladek, and Jürgen Unützer, *Fixing Behavioral Health Care in America: A National Call for Measurement-Based Care in the Delivery of Behavioral Health Services*, Chicago: Kennedy Forum, 2015.

Fortney, John C., Jürgen Unützer, Glenda Wrenn, Jeffrey M. Pyne, G. Richard Smith, Michael Schoenbaum, and Henry T. Harbin, "A Tipping Point for Measurement-Based Care," *Psychiatric Services,* Vol. 68, No. 2, February 2017, pp. 179–188.

Fox, Annie B., Eric C. Meyer, and Dawne Vogt, "Attitudes About the VA Health-Care Setting, Mental Illness, and Mental Health Treatment and Their Relationship with VA Mental Health Service Use Among Female and Male OEF/OIF Veterans," *Psychological Services,* Vol. 12, No. 1, February 2015, pp. 49–58.

Garcia, Hector A., Erin P. Finley, Norma Ketchum, Matthew Jakupcak, Albana Dassori, and Stephanie C. Reyes, "A Survey of Perceived Barriers and Attitudes Toward Mental Health Care Among OEF/OIF Veterans at VA Outpatient Mental Health Clinics," *Military Medicine,* Vol. 179, No. 3, March 2014, pp. 273–278.

George W. Bush Institute, "Veteran Wellness Alliance," webpage, undated. As of September 8, 2020:
https://www.bushcenter.org/veteran-wellness/index.html

Hamblen, Jessica L., Sonya B. Norman, Jeffrey H. Sonis, Andrea J. Phelps, Jonathan I. Bisson, Vanessa D. Nunes, Odette Megnin-Viggars, David Forbes, David S. Riggs, and Paula P. Schnurr, "A Guide to Guidelines for the Treatment of Posttraumatic Stress Disorder in Adults: An Update," *Psychotherapy,* Vol. 56, No. 3, September 2019, pp. 359–373.

Hamm, William G., Virginia T. Betts, Dennis M. Duffy, Frank A. Fairbanks, Thomas L. Garthwaite, Donald F. Kettl, Bernard D. Rostker, and Daniel L. Skoler, *After Yellow Ribbons: Providing Veteran-Centered Services,* Washington, D.C.: National Academy of Public Administration, October 2008. As of September 8, 2020:
https://www.napawash.org/uploads/Academy_Studies/08-14.pdf

Hepner, Kimberly A., Stephanie Brooks Holliday, Jessica L. Sousa, and Terri Tanielian, *User Guide for the Training in Psychotherapy (TIP) Tool 2.0,* Santa Monica, Calif.: RAND Corporation, TL-306-1-MTF, 2019. As of September 8, 2020:
https://www.rand.org/pubs/tools/TL306-1.html

Hepner, Kimberly A., Elizabeth M. Sloss, Carol P. Roth, Heather Krull, Susan M. Paddock, Shaela Moen, Martha J. Timmer, and Harold Alan Pincus, *Quality of Care for PTSD and Depression in the Military Health System: Phase I Report,* Santa Monica, Calif.: RAND Corporation, RR-978-OSD, 2016. As of September 8, 2020:
https://www.rand.org/pubs/research_reports/RR978.html

Hoge, Charles W., Carl A. Castro, Stephen C. Messer, Dennis McGurk, Dave I. Cotting, and Robert L. Koffman, "Combat Duty in Iraq and Afghanistan, Mental Health Problems, and Barriers to Care," *New England Journal of Medicine,* Vol. 351, No. 1, July 1, 2004, pp. 13–22.

Horvat, Lidia, Dell Horey, Panayiota Romios, and John Kis-Rigo, "Cultural Competence Education for Health Professionals," *Cochrane Database of Systematic Reviews,* Vol. 5, No. 5, May 2014.

Hussey, Peter S., Jeanne S. Ringel, Sangeeta C. Ahluwalia, Rebecca Anhang Price, Christine Buttorff, Thomas W. Concannon, Susan L. Lovejoy, Grant R. Martsolf, Robert S. Rudin, Dana Schultz, et al., *Resources and Capabilities of the Department of Veterans Affairs to Provide Timely and Accessible Care to Veterans,* Santa Monica, Calif.: RAND Corporation, RR-1165/2-VA, 2015. As of September 8, 2020: https://www.rand.org/pubs/research_reports/RR1165z2.html

Institute for Patient- and Family-Centered Care, *Advancing the Practice of Patient- and Family-Centered Care in Primary Care and Other Ambulatory Settings: How to Get Started,* Bethesda, Md., 2016. As of September 8. 2020: https://www.ipfcc.org/resources/GettingStarted-AmbulatoryCare.pdf

Institute of Medicine, *Crossing the Quality Chasm: A New Health System for the 21st Century,* Washington, D.C.: National Academies Press, 2001a.

———, *Envisioning the National Health Care Quality Report,* Washington, D.C.: National Academies Press, 2001b.

———, *Treatment for Posttraumatic Stress Disorder in Military and Veteran Populations: Final Assessment,* Washington, D.C.: National Academies Press, 2014.

International Society for Traumatic Stress Studies, *Posttraumatic Stress Disorder Prevention and Treatment Guidelines: Methodology and Recommendations,* Oakbrook Terrace, Ill., October 30, 2017.

IOM—*See* Institute of Medicine.

Joosten, E. A. G., L. DeFuentes-Merillas, G. H. de Weert, T. Sensky, C. P. F. van der Staak, and C. A. J. de Jong, "Systematic Review of the Effects of Shared Decision-Making on Patient Satisfaction, Treatment Adherence and Health Status," *Psychotherapy and Psychosomatics,* Vol. 77, No. 4, May 2008, pp. 219–226.

Jorge, Ricardo E., Laura Acion, Debora I. Burin, and Robert G. Robinson, "Sertraline for Preventing Mood Disorders Following Traumatic Brain Injury: A Randomized Clinical Trial," *JAMA Psychiatry,* Vol. 73, No. 10, October 2016, pp. 1041–1047.

Kearney, Lisa K., Laura O. Wray, Katherine M. Dollar, and Paul R. King, "Establishing Measurement-based Care in Integrated Primary Care: Monitoring Clinical Outcomes Over Time," *Journal of Clinical Psychology in Medical Settings,* Vol. 22, No. 4, December 2015, pp. 213–227.

Kitchiner, Neil J., Catrin Lewis, Neil P. Roberts, and Jonathan I. Bisson, "Active Duty and Ex-Serving Military Personnel with Post-Traumatic Stress Disorder Treated with Psychological Therapies: Systematic Review and Meta-Analysis," *European Journal of Psychotraumatology*, Vol. 10, No. 1, 2019, article 1684226.

Klerman, Gerald L., Myrna M. Weissman, Bruce J. Rounsaville, and Eve S. Chevron, *Interpersonal Psychotherapy of Depression*, New York: Basic Books, 1984.

Knaup, Carina, Markus Koesters, Dorothea Schoefer, Thomas Becker, and Bernd Puschner, "Effect of Feedback of Treatment Outcome in Specialist Mental Healthcare: Meta-Analysis," *British Journal of Psychiatry,* Vol. 195, No. 1, July 2009, pp. 15–22.

Kokorelias, Kristina M., Monique A. M. Gignac, Gary Naglie, and Jill I. Cameron, "Towards a Universal Model of Family Centered Care: A Scoping Review," *BMC Health Services Research,* Vol. 19, No. 1, 2019, article 564.

Kroenke, Kurt, Robert L. Spitzer, and Janet B. W. Williams, "The PHQ-9: Validity of a Brief Depression Severity Measure," *Journal of General Internal Medicine,* Vol. 16, No. 9, September 2001, pp. 606–613.

Lambert, Michael J., Jason L. Whipple, Eric J. Hawkins, David A. Vermeersch, Stevan L. Nielsen, and David W. Smart, "Is It Time for Clinicians to Routinely Track Patient Outcome? A Meta-Analysis," *Clinical Psychology: Science and Practice,* Vol. 10, No. 3, September 2003, pp. 288–301.

Lavin, Peggy, Lynn Berry, and Scott Williams, "Measurement-Based Care in Behavioral Health," webinar slides, Oakbrook Terrace, Ill.: Joint Commission, Accreditation Behavioral Health Care, 2017.

Lewis, Cara C., Meredith Boyd, Ajeng Puspitasari, Elena Navarro, Jacqueline Howard, Hannah Kassab, Mira Hoffman, Kelli Scott, Aaron Lyon, Susan Douglas, Greg Simon, and Kurt Kroenke, "Implementing Measurement-Based Care in Behavioral Health: A Review," *JAMA Psychiatry,* Vol. 76, No. 3, March 2019, pp. 324–335.

Lumba-Brown, Angela, Keith Owen Yeates, Kelly Sarmiento, Matthew J. Breiding, Tamara M. Haegerich, Gerard A. Gioia, Michael Turner, Edward C. Benzel, Stacy J. Suskauer, Christopher C. Giza, et al., "Centers for Disease Control and Prevention Guideline on the Diagnosis and Management of Mild Traumatic Brain Injury Among Children," *JAMA Pediatrics,* Vol. 172, No. 11, November 2018a, article e182853.

———, "Diagnosis and Management of Mild Traumatic Brain Injury in Children: A Systematic Review," *JAMA Pediatrics,* Vol. 172, No. 11, November 2018b, article e182847.

Marshall, Shawn, Mark Bayley, Scott McCullagh, Lindsay Berrigan, Lisa Fischer, Donna Ouchterlony, C. Rockwell, Diana Velikokja, *Guideline for Concussion/Mild Traumatic Brain Injury and Prolonged Symptoms*, 3rd ed. for adults 18+ years of age, Toronto, Canada: Ontario Neurotrauma Foundation, 2018. As of September 8, 2020:
https://braininjuryguidelines.org/concussion

McCrory, Paul, Willem Meeuwisse, Jiří Dvorak, Mark Aubry, Julian Bailes, Steven Broglio, Robert C. Cantu, David Cassidy, Ruben J. Echemendia, Rudy J. Castellani, et al., "Consensus Statement on Concussion in Sport— The 5th International Conference on Concussion in Sport Held in Berlin, October 2016," *British Journal of Sports Medicine,* Vol. 51, No. 11, June 2017, pp. 838–847.

Meyer, Erik, Brian W. Writer, and William Brim, "The Importance of Military Cultural Competence," *Current Psychiatry Reports*, Vol. 18, No. 3, March 2016, article 26.

National Institute for Health and Care Excellence, *Post-Traumatic Stress Disorder: NICE Guideline*, London, December 5, 2018.

Park, Stephanie G., Marisa Derman, Lisa B. Dixon, Clayton H. Brown, Elizabeth A. Klingaman, Li Juan Fang, Deborah R. Medoff, and Julie Kreyenbuhl, "Factors Associated with Shared Decision-Making Preferences Among Veterans with Serious Mental Illness," *Psychiatric Services*, Vol. 65, No. 12, December 1, 2014, pp. 1409–1413.

Penchansky, Roy, and J. William Thomas, "The Concept of Access: Definition and Relationship to Consumer Satisfaction," *Medical Care,* Vol. 19, No. 2, February 1981, pp. 127–140.

Pizer, Steven D., and Julia C. Prentice, "What Are the Consequences of Waiting for Health Care in the Veteran Population?" *Journal of General Internal Medicine,* Vol. 26, Suppl. 2, November 2011, pp. 676–682.

Polinder, Suzanne, Maryse C. Cnossen, Ruben G. L. Real, Amra Covic, Anastasia Gorbunova, Daphne C. Voormolen, Christina L. Master, Juanita A. Haagsma, Ramon Diaz-Arrastia, and Nicole von Steinbuechel, "A Multidimensional Approach to Post-Concussion Symptoms in Mild Traumatic Brain Injury," *Frontiers in Neurology,* December 19, 2018, article 1113.

Potter, Sebastian D. S., Richard G. Brown, and Simon Fleminger, "Randomised, Waiting List Controlled Trial of Cognitive-Behavioural Therapy for Persistent Postconcussional Symptoms After Predominantly Mild–Moderate Traumatic Brain Injury," *Journal of Neurology, Neurosurgery and Psychiatry,* Vol. 87, No. 10, October 2016, pp. 1075–1083.

Prentice, Julia C., and Steven D. Pizer, "Delayed Access to Health Care and Mortality," *Health Services Research,* Vol. 42, No. 2, April 2007, pp. 644–662.

Sackett, David L., William M. C. Rosenberg, J. A. Muir Gray, R. Brian Haynes, and W. Scott Richardson, "Evidence Based Medicine: What It Is and What It Isn't," *British Medical Journal*, Vol. 312, No. 7023, January 13, 1996, pp. 71–72.

Santana, Maria-Jose, and David Feeny, "Framework to Assess the Effects of Using Patient-Reported Outcome Measures in Chronic Care Management," *Quality of Life Research*, Vol. 23, No. 5, June 2014, pp. 1505–1513.

Scott, Kelli, and Cara C. Lewis, "Using Measurement-Based Care to Enhance Any Treatment," *Cognitive and Behavioral Practice*, Vol. 22, No. 1, February 2015, pp. 49–59.

Shay, L. Aubree, and Jennifer Elston Lafata, "Where Is the Evidence? A Systematic Review of Shared Decision Making and Patient Outcomes," *Medical Decision Making*, Vol. 35, No. 1, 2015, pp. 114–131.

Shimokawa, Kenichi, Michael J. Lambert, and David W. Smart, "Enhancing Treatment Outcome of Patients at Risk of Treatment Failure: Meta-Analytic and Mega-Analytic Review of a Psychotherapy Quality Assurance System," *Journal of Consulting and Clinical Psychology*, Vol. 78, No. 3, June 2010, pp. 298–311.

Silverberg, Noah D., Ann-Christine Duhaime, and Mary Alexis Iaccarino, "Mild Traumatic Brain Injury in 2019–2020," *Journal of the American Medical Association*, Vol. 323, No. 2, January 14, 2020, pp. 177–178.

Spitzer, Robert L., Kurt Kroenke, Janet B. W. Williams, and Bernd Löwe, "A Brief Measure for Assessing Generalized Anxiety Disorder: The GAD-7," *Archives of Internal Medicine*, Vol. 166, No. 10, May 22, 2006, pp. 1092–1097.

Stacey, Dawn, France Légaré, Krystina Lewis, Michael J. Barry, Carol L. Bennett, Karen B. Eden, Margaret Holmes-Rovner, Hilary Llewellyn-Thomas, Anne Lyddiatt, Richard Thomson, and Lyndal Trevena, "Decision Aids for People Facing Health Treatment or Screening Decisions," *Cochrane Database of Systematic Reviews*, Vol. 4, No. 4, 2017.

Steenkamp, Maria M., Brett T. Litz, Charles W. Hoge, and Charles R. Marmar, "Psychotherapy for Military-Related PTSD: A Review of Randomized Clinical Trials," *Journal of the American Medical Association*, Vol. 314, No. 5, August 4, 2015, pp. 489–500.

Steenkamp, Maria M., Brett T. Litz, and Charles R. Marmar, "First-Line Psychotherapies for Military-Related PTSD," *Journal of the American Medical Association*, Vol. 323, No. 7, February 18, 2020, pp. 656–657.

Tanielian, Terri, Coreen Farris, Caroline Batka, Carrie M. Farmer, Eric Robinson, Charles C. Engel, Michael W. Robbins, and Lisa H. Jaycox, *Ready to Serve: Community-Based Provider Capacity to Deliver Culturally Competent, Quality Mental Health Care to Veterans and Their Families*, Santa Monica, Calif.: RAND Corporation, RR-806-UNHF, 2014. As of September 8, 2020: https://www.rand.org/pubs/research_reports/RR806.html

Tanielian, Terri, and Lisa H. Jaycox, eds., *Invisible Wounds of War: Psychological and Cognitive Injuries, Their Consequences, and Services to Assist Recovery*, Santa Monica, Calif.: RAND Corporation, MG-720-CCF, 2008. As of September 8, 2020:
https://www.rand.org/pubs/monographs/MG720.html

Teich, Judith, Mir M. Ali, Sean Lynch, and Ryan Mutter, "Utilization of Mental Health Services by Veterans Living in Rural Areas," *Journal of Rural Health*, Vol. 33, No. 3, June 2017, pp. 297–304.

Trivedi, Ranak B., Edward P. Post, Haili Sun, Andrew Pomerantz, Andrew J. Saxon, John D. Piette, Charles Maynard, Bruce Arnow, Idamay Curtis, Stephan D. Fihn, and Karin Nelson, "Prevalence, Comorbidity, and Prognosis of Mental Health Among US Veterans," *American Journal of Public Health*, Vol. 105, No. 12, December 2015, pp. 2564–2569.

U.S. Department of Veterans Affairs, "Access and Quality in VA Healthcare," webpage, undated. As of September 8, 2020:
https://www.accesstocare.va.gov

———, "Measurement-Based Care (MBC) in Mental Health Initiative," press release, May 2016. As of September 8, 2020:
https://www.mirecc.va.gov/visn4/docs/MBCinMHInitiative.pdf

———, "Evidence-Based Practice Program," webpage, last updated May 14, 2019. As of September 8, 2020:
https://www.va.gov/HEALTHCAREEXCELLENCE/about/organization/examples/evidence-based-practice-program.asp

U.S. Department of Veterans Affairs and U.S. Department of Defense, *VA/DoD Clinical Practice Guideline for the Management of Concussion—Mild Traumatic Brain Injury*, version 2.0, Washington, D.C., 2016.

———, *VA/DoD Clinical Practice Guideline for the Management of Posttraumatic Stress Disorder and Acute Stress Disorder*, version 3.0, Washington, D.C., 2017.

VA—*See* U.S. Department of Veterans Affairs.

VA/DoD—*See* U.S. Department of Veterans Affairs and U.S. Department of Defense.

Weathers, F. W., B. T. Litz, T. M. Keane, P. A. Palmieri, B. P. Marx, and P. P. Schnurr, *The PTSD Checklist for DSM-5 (PCL-5)*, Washington, D.C.: U.S. Department of Veterans Affairs, 2013.

World Health Organization, *Guidelines for the Management of Conditions Specifically Related to Stress*, Geneva, Switzerland, 2013.

Wounded Warrior Project, "Warrior Care Network," webpage, undated. As of September 8, 2020:
https://www.woundedwarriorproject.org/programs/warrior-care-network

Wray, Laura O., Mona J. Ritchie, David W. Oslin, and Gregory P. Beehler, "Enhancing Implementation of Measurement-Based Mental Health Care in Primary Care: A Mixed-Methods Randomized Effectiveness Evaluation of Implementation Facilitation," *BMC Health Services Research,* Vol. 18, No. 1, 2018, article 753.